ANTI INFLAMMATORY & ALKALINE DIET

FOR BEGINNERS

A Natural Path For Life-Long Health | How To Detox Your Body And Reduce Inflammation The Quick & Easy Way

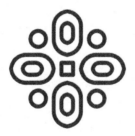

Serena Stewart

CONTENTS

INTRODUCTION

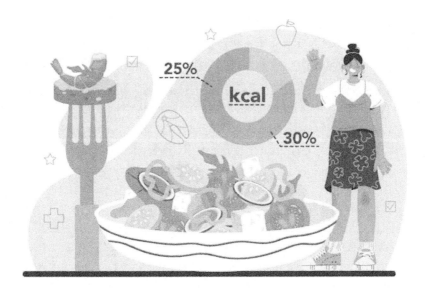

The relationship between healthy eating and health is very close: in fact, it is scientifically proven that health is built at the table, based on the food we eat. That's why this book aims to be a vademecum for a natural, balanced and clean eating.

Following a healthy diet brings with it countless benefits, if followed consistently and understood as a lifestyle: Over time, it is the everyday practice of good habits that make a difference. The necessity of a varied and balanced diet cannot be overstated, since this ensures that all of the body's vital nutrients are being consumed (carbohydrates, proteins, fats, vitamins and minerals). Eating a healthy diet not only prevents disease and extends life expectancy, but also improves one's mood, energy, and overall well-being. It is necessary to have the right balance in food choices: constantly depriving oneself and giving up foods considered "banned" leads to temptation, consequent giving in perceived as failure, and thus a vicious cycle is generated, which progressively distances one from one's goal. The truth is that there are no "forbidden" foods that must be eliminated, as neither are there any "miracle" healthy foods, but there is the right balance, made up of healthy daily food choices alternating with opportunities for gluttony. Healthy eating should not be interpreted as a means to solve, but to prevent. It therefore turns out to be essential to follow a healthy and proper diet in all age groups:

- From birth to adolescence, nutrition should be understood as real nutrition, necessary to promote growth and proper development. The basics of healthy eating should be conveyed to the youngest: how to take in wholesome foods, follow their seasonality, avoid junk food, involve them in the choices and preparation of meals, because these simple habits once acquired will be maintained for the rest of life;

- From the third to the fourth age, to prevent numerous diseases, such as overweight and obesity, conditions that threaten the Western world today, so much so that there is talk of globesity (a term coined to indicate a true global emergency). Worsening this situation is another predominant factor: *sedentariness*. The WHO estimates that about 41 percent of Americans do not engage in any kind of physical activity during the week, and this increases the risk of chronic diseases.

In this sense, the importance of following a healthy diet, together with the proper performance of physical activity, can help prevent numerous diseases, including the aforementioned obesity, a risk factor for:

- **Cardiovascular disease:** due to a diet high in saturated fat and low in fiber, it promotes the development of atherosclerosis;

- **Type 2 diabetes:** associated with numerous complications such as cardiovascular disease, kidney disease, diabetic vasculopathy and blindness;

- **Osteoporosis**: resulting from a 'diet low in calcium and vitamin D, increases the risk of fractures and reduces the quality of life;

- **Gastrointestinal issues;**

- **Autoimmune and inflammatory diseases:** especially during this sensitive period, healthy eating allows the immune system to be fortified.

Proper nutrition means not only the quality of what we eat at the table, but also when and how many times a day we eat. Meals mark our day and allow us to create a healthy routine that is also metabolic. Hence the importance of not skipping meals and dividing the day into three main meals (breakfast, lunch, dinner) plus two snacks. The time to eat the meal is also important, hence the need to chew the food slowly not only because digestion begins in the first part of the digestive canal i.e., in the mouth, but also because the satiety stimulus is delayed and comes about 20 minutes after the meal is finished. Last factor is conviviality: sharing mealtime with one's family members from an early age gives food a different value and puts one in a position to appreciate what one eats more. From an early age, mealtime is a key time for assimilating healthy eating habits, hygiene rules and social rules.

It only remains for me to welcome you to the health and food awareness journey contained in the pages that follow. I hope you will gain more than a few insights to start your new-tritious lifestyle on the right foot.

Have a good read,

Serena Stewart

THE IMPORTANCE OF NUTRITION

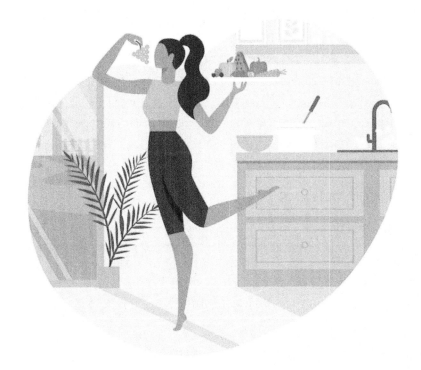

Food. We all love it. We are literally unable to do without it. But did you know that not all the food we put in our mouths is really nutritious? In reality, many "comfort foods" (chips, ice cream, sweets, and other industrially processed meals)

don't provide much nourishment.Sure, they taste good, but from a nutrient standpoint they are not much! So what if we can't get the nutrients we need from food? Can we take advantage of other sources? And why is nutrition important anyway? Take your time reading this chapter since it will answer all of your questions and more!

QUALITY IS A MUST

If you want to live a long, healthy and happy life there is first of all a need for your nutrition to be adequate. It is hard to enjoy life if you are weak and don't feel 100% all the time. Good nutrition allows the body to work, grow and thrive! What exactly does "good nutrition" mean? Well, first of all, it means eating more of the right foods in the right quantities. By "right" foods, we mean foods rich in nutrients from a variety of groups, for example:ù

- Protein-rich foods
- Cereals
- Vegetables
- Fruits

When you refuel your body with all these healthy foods, it drastically decreases the likelihood of stuffing yourself with calorie-rich but nutrient-poor junk food and drinks. Unfortunately, the food choices of modern life almost make it seem that healthy eating is optional. We tend to be lazy when it comes to eating because of our hectic lives. Many prefer to munch on what is immediately ready and available, no matter how unhealthy it is. Junk food and fast food is cheap and accessible for everyone. There is no need to prepare anything: just pay for it and you are ready to eat.

On the other hand, healthy and nutritious food is definitely more expensive. It also requires preparation, which means it takes time to cook it and make it tasty. Unfortunately, many people cannot afford either the money or the time to prepare nutritious food for themselves, so they end up stuffing themselves with junk food.

BENEFITS OF CONSCIOUS EATING

If you've spent the most of your life eating an unhealthy diet, you'll have a lot of work to do to get back on track. Stopping the poor habits you've had your whole life will be difficult, but it's critical that you begin as soon as possible (even today, if feasible) for the sake of your health! To give you a sense of how essential good eating is, here are ten of the most significant advantages:

1) NUTRIENTS CONTRIBUTE TO THE BODY'S VITAL FUNCTIONS

Nutrients from the food we eat promote the growth, maintenance, and repair of our body's cells and tissues. For example, vitamin A is necessary for us to see well, and vitamin D helps maintain a healthy immune system. As you can imagine, a deficiency of essential nutrients can lead to disastrous health consequences.

2) IMPROVES CARDIOVASCULAR HEALTH

A sedentary lifestyle combined with poor diet may contribute to the development of cardiovascular disease. Avoid foods with a high concentration of trans and saturated fats. These fats are deemed "bad" because they enhance "bad" cholesterol (LDL) levels while decreasing good cholesterol levels (HDL).

3) BETTER NUTRITION MEANS BETTER IMMUNITY

We need stronger immunity now, more than ever, in the middle of a worldwide epidemic. Consuming healthy meals can assist your body in fighting viruses, germs, and other pathogens that you may come into touch with.

4) IT KEEPS YOU FIT AND IMPROVES YOUR WEIGHT

What you see on the scale is a good indicator of whether you are eating well or not. This is because malnutrition can take many forms: malnourished individuals can be thin and underweight, or overweight or obese. By improving your diet, the needle on the scale will move up or down, depending on where your body needs to be from a weight perspective.

5) IT GIVES YOU A BETTER APPEARANCE

Good nutrition also has an impact on your outward appearance. For example, if you eat foods rich in healthy fats, such as oily fish, avocados, nuts, and vegetables, you'll be more likely to have brighter skin and be less prone to acne.

6) HELPS SLOW THE AGING PROCESS

Sooner or later, we all get old. But a healthy diet can slow down the aging process! You won't have to spend a lot of money on facial massages and skin-improving treatments-you only need to start eating a light, healthy diet to start seeing improvements.

7) ALLOWS HEALTHY PREGNANCY

Regardless of your gender, if you want to have children someday, then you need to be healthy. Otherwise, your fertility may suffer. Also, women are much more likely to carry a pregnancy to term (giving birth to a healthy, full-term baby) if they themselves are healthy.

8) IMPROVES MENTAL HEALTH

Yes, the food we eat affects mental health as a whole. For example, did you know that omega-3 fatty acids promote brain health? Omega-3 is abundant in oily fish, so be sure to include it in your diet. If you're not too fond of fish and/or shellfish, why not try supplementing with our Ultra Pure Fish Oil with Triglycerides and Omega-3?

9) REDUCES THE RISK OF CHRONIC DISEASE

Living with a chronic disease is not pleasant, especially when its symptoms become unmanageable. Fortunately, eating healthy can reduce your risk of developing chronic diseases. But what if you are already suffering from it?

A healthy diet can help you manage your symptoms. For example, if you have type 2 diabetes, if you avoid eating foods high in carbohydrates that raise insulin levels, then you may be able to manage your diabetes.

10) PROPER NUTRITION INCREASES ENERGY LEVELS

All you need to do is eat the right way to experience a new sense of strength and energy. This is because a healthy diet indicates that you are supplying your body with energy-filled macronutrients, such as carbohydrates, protein, and unsaturated fat (i.e., the "good" kind of fat).

THE ESSENTIAL NUTRIENTS

Protein, carbs, fat, water, vitamins, and minerals are the six fundamental elements that the body need to operate correctly. They are classified into two groups: macronutrients and micronutrients.

1) Macronutrients

Our bodies need macronutrients in large quantities (usually measured in grams). These nutrients give the body energy. There are four types of macronutrients:

- Protein
- Carbohydrates
- Fats
- Water

Here is a summary with the best food sources of macronutrients:

- **Protein:** Shellfish, meat, poultry, eggs, nuts, dairy products
- **Carbohydrates:** Whole grains, whole wheat flour, potatoes, legumes, corn, beans, fiber-rich fruits, starchy vegetables
- **Fats:** Oily fish, eggs, nuts, seeds, avocados, olive oil, peanut oil, cheese, dairy products
- **Water:** Drinking water, watermelons, oranges, coconut

2) Micronutrients

Ours requires smaller amounts of micronutrients. They are normally measured in milligrams or micrograms. There are two types of micronutrients:

Vitamins-there are 13 vitamins

● The 8 B-complex vitamins: B1, B2, B3, B5, B6, B7, B9 and B12.

● The vitamins A, C, D, E and K

Mineral salts

● Most important minerals: you need more than small traces of these minerals. Some examples: calcium, magnesium, sodium and phosphorus.

● Trace minerals: they are still needed but huge amounts are not needed. Among them: iron, manganese, zinc, copper, iodine, selenium and fluoride.

Here is a table with the best food sources of micronutrients:

● Vitamin A: Liver, fish, carrots, broccoli, eggplant, fortified cereals.

● Vitamin C: Chili, kale, broccoli, oranges, lemons, strawberries.

● Vitamin D: Liver, salmon, red meat, cod liver oil, egg yolk, fortified foods.

● Vitamin E: Almonds, sunflower seeds, hazelnuts, peanuts, avocados.

● Vitamin K: Black cabbage, spinach, lettuce, broccoli, cauliflower, cabbage.

● Vitamin B: Liver, eggs, shellfish, dairy products, seeds, poultry, meat.

- Mineral Salts: Dried fruits, seeds, animal organs, eggs, beans, shellfish, vegetables.

Are you ready to take charge of your diet now that you understand why excellent nutrition is so important? Begin your road to healthy eating by making a tiny sacrifice: clean out your cupboard by tossing away any junk food. Natural and less processed food can be substituted. It's true that saying it is easier than doing it. To be honest, saying it is easier than doing it. You'll learn more about what it means to eat healthfully in the following chapters.

CHAPTER 2

THE ALKALINE DIET

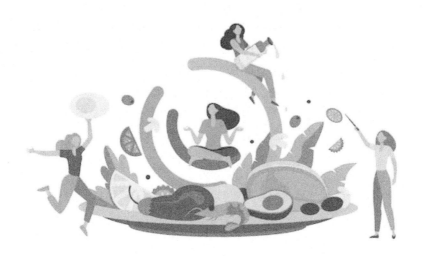

Alkaline diet, you have all heard of this dietary regimen at least once and may have even experienced it firsthand. Let's learn more about how the alkaline diet works, what you can eat and what foods you should limit. Aimed not so much at weight loss as at increasing the body's well-being and vitality, the alkaline diet or alkalizing diet was devised by Robert O. Young, a naturopath and nutritionist. It is based on some specific assumptions that cannot be separated from knowledge of such a parameter as pH and the importance it has within our bodies.

What is pH? - pH refers to the unit of measurement by which we determine whether an organic liquid (blood, urine, etc.) is acidic or basic, that is, whether, according to a scale ranging from 0 to 14, it has a value lower than 7 (acidic), higher (alkaline) or even (neutral). When acidity is found, it means that there is a high presence of hydrogen ions (pH in fact stands for Potentia Hidrogens) within the body and this, in the long run, can lead to the appearance of various disorders including diseases due to cell degeneration.

The accumulation of acid within our bodies can originate from a variety of causes: poor diet, use of medications, bad habits such as smoking and excessive alcohol consumption, stress, sedentary lifestyle and more. Many of us, therefore, are at risk of acidosis, which is when it can come in handy to follow, at least for a period, an alkaline diet.

BASIC PRINCIPLES

So, what does the so-called alkaline diet involve? Can this diet regimen really help us lose weight, reduce inflammation and improve health? It is an eating regimen that harnesses the power of certain plant-based foods with strong anti-inflammatory qualities to promote better health but also to promote weight loss. Let's find out how it works and then see a 7-day menu suitable for following it.

The theory behind the alkaline diet is to divide different foods into acidic or alkaline, taking as a reference point the pH scale ranging from 0 to 14. If the value of the individual food is lower than 7, we are in the presence of an acidic food; if higher, an alkaline food. Therefore, it is believed that some foods, such as meat, wheat, refined sugar and processed foods, are responsible for our bodies producing acids, which is bad for our health.

In fact, foods high in sugar and fat slightly increase the acidity of the blood, and this promotes inflammation within our bodies. In response, the body is forced to filter minerals from the bones and organs to restore the correct pH value, which is 7.4.

FOODS TO EAT

The alkalizing diet is based mainly on the use of vegetables and fruits, some grains and legumes, nuts and oil seeds, sprouts, and essential fatty acids such as those found in flax oil and olive oil (omega 3 and omega 6). Among the absolute most alkalizing foods is grapes; it is no coincidence that this fruit often appears in detoxification diets; there is even a purifying system that involves eating only grapes for one or more days.

Other foods with alkalizing power include: beets, turnips, carrots, radishes, cabbage, cauliflower, broccoli, spinach, Swiss chard, garlic, lemons, cucumbers, celery, apples, carrots, dried figs, bean sprouts, lettuce, avocados and mushrooms. Condiments with alkalizing power include ginger, chili peppers, curry, sage, rosemary, cumin seeds, and fennel seeds. In contrast, the only alkalizing grains (or cereal-like grains) are quinoa, millet and amaranth. To recap when following an alkaline or alkalizing diet you need to increase your intake of:

- grapes
- beets
- turnips
- carrots
- radishes
- cabbage
- cauliflower
- broccoli
- spinach
- chard
- garlic
- lemon
- cucumbers
- celery
- apples
- figs
- bean sprouts
- lettuce
- avocado
- mushrooms
- millet
- quinoa

- amaranth
- ginger
- chili
- curry
- sage
- rosemary
- fennel seeds
- cumin seeds
- extra virgin olive oil
- linseed oil
- nuts and oil seeds

FOODS TO AVOID

There are several alkalizing foods, but this does not mean that you should only eat those all the time. Excessively alkalizing the body can also bring disadvantages. As always, one must know how to use the right medium and, if possible, avoid DIY but rely on the advice of an expert who will best calibrate on the individual case the best diet to follow.

Rather than foods to avoid, it would be better to talk about foods to limit when you need to alkalize your body. Foods that contain yeast and sugar, those that are refined, processed, microwaved but also fermented are considered acidifying. Grains are almost all acidifying among them: wheat, spelt, oats, rice, rye, corn, barley and all their derivatives, including bread and pasta. Some legumes are also acidifying among these are chickpeas, white beans and lentils. Among animal proteins: meat, but also fish such as cod, salmon as well as eggs, milk and cheese. Sweeteners to limit include sugar and honey. To recapitulate to limit are:

- yeast
- sugar
- refined or processed foods
- cooked or microwaved foods
- fermented foods
- wheat
- spelt
- oats
- rye
- rice
- corn
- barley
- bread and pasta
- chickpeas
- white beans
- lentils
- meat

- fish

- eggs

- cheese and milk

- honey

As we have already specified the foods listed above are not necessarily to be eliminated completely, the important thing is to know how to find the right food balance while avoiding the excessive formation of acids within our bodies If, for example, one realizes that one's diet is too unbalanced in favor of acidifying foods, one can begin to include more alkalizing foods on a daily basis. Generally, however, the alkaline diet recommends that you should prefer 70-80% alkaline foods every day as opposed to 20-30% acidic foods. Vegetables should always be eaten at least partially raw.

TOP 10 ALKALINE FOODS TO EAT EVERY DAY

In the alkaline diet, an acidifying effect on the body is one of the characteristic difficulties of the current diet, which consists mostly of packaged, refined and processed foods and animal protein and sugar. This has health effects that can lead to inflammatory disorders and cancer. As a result, it would be beneficial to include more and more foods that can help restore the body's pH to a more alkaline state. To be sure, the foods advocated (all from the plant kingdom) are healthy, but even if you don't believe in this theory, which critics say has no scientific foundation, you have to admit that their properties have been confirmed by numerous studies measuring their characteristics and benefits to the human body. Because of this, we suggest including them on a regular basis and varying your servings based on the time of year and your own preferences.

TUBERS AND ROOTS

The body is alkaline when it consumes beets, turnips, radishes, and other edible roots and tubers. Aside from their nutritional value, the minerals and fiber they contain help

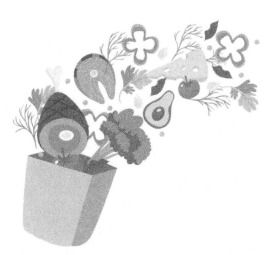

keep the body healthy as a whole. A trickle of extra virgin olive oil may be drizzled over them after they've been cooked or eaten raw or even steamed.

CRUCIFERS

The beneficial effects of crucifers (the whole family of cabbage and broccoli) are now renowned. In addition to shifting the body's pH to mild alkalinity they strengthen the immune system, improve digestion, and have also been credited with gifts in the prevention of certain cancers. When in season, they can be eaten every day, the variety in fact is very wide and one can choose from broccoli, cauliflower, kale, greens, etc.

GREEN LEAFY VEGETABLES

Raw or steamed, green leafy vegetables are among the healthiest meals you can eat. Alternate between raw and steaming servings based on the season. Spinach and chard are excellent examples of foods that help maintain a healthy acid-base balance in the body. Fiber, minerals, and vitamins are all present in these foods as well, making them beneficial to our health on a daily basis.

GARLIC

People who want to maintain good health should consume a lot of garlic because of its many beneficial properties. Garlic is not only alkalizing, but it also acts as a natural antibiotic, strengthens the heart and immune system, reduces inflammation and free radicals, and aids in the body's detoxification process. Since it is cheap and readily available, it can be called a superfood in every sense of the word.

LEMONS

Lemons have a naturally acidic pH due to the citric acid they contain, so referring to them as an alkalizing meal may sound unusual at first. Once the lemon is in the body, the alkalizing effect begins, especially if it is eaten with water on an empty stomach in the morning. One can get a slew of benefits, including improved digestion, better liver function, a boost to the immune system, and weight loss. A person's energy and vitality can be seen in the early hours of the morning as a result of all this.

CUCUMBER

Water content of cucumbers can reach up to 95%, making them a particularly valuable alkalizing vegetable. It's no coincidence that this vegetable's peak season is in the summer, when it's packed with antioxidants, vitamins, and minerals, all of which make it an excellent source of hydration. Juicing cucumbers with other vegetables and fruits is a terrific way to eat them, but they may also be eaten raw in salads.

SEDAR

Celery, like cucumber, is an alkaline vegetable with a high water content that is commonly used in soups and stir-fries, but it is best consumed raw in a pinzimonio or juiced to get the most out of its qualities. A good source of vitamin C, celery is also a wonderful choice for individuals who wish to lose weight because it is low in calories and diuretic, making it ideal for those who are trying to slim down.

APPLES

Apples are alkalizing, as are most fruits, and they offer the body with fiber, which is crucial for intestinal health, as well as vitamins, minerals, and other elements. In order to eat them whole, it is critical that they are organically grown, as the peel is the most nutrient-dense section.

AVOCADO

Because of its unique characteristics, the avocado truly is a gift from the gods. In spite of its high fat content, it is a good source of important fatty acids such as Omega 3, and when ingested in moderation, it does not contribute to weight gain. This fruit is rich in minerals, vitamins, and antioxidants, as well as a pH alkalizer.

GRAPES

Grapes are also well-known for their alkalizing qualities, which have been documented. In order to be hydrated and healthy, our bodies need the antioxidants, minerals, vitamins, and resveratrol that are present in a wide variety of fruits and vegetables. The grape treatment is a well-known method for balancing the pH of the body and purifying and detoxifying it. It entails ingesting only grape juice or whole grapes for 1-2 or 3 days.

THE SECRET TO BALANCING THE BODY'S PH

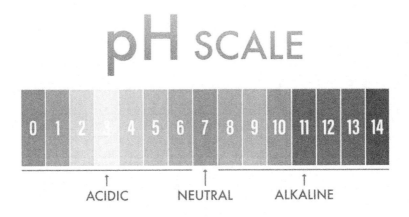

pH SCALE

ACIDIC   NEUTRAL   ALKALINE

Acidifying foods and alkalizing foods. What foods to choose in order to rebalance the pH of our body? Going in search of information regarding natural nutrition, it may happen to encounter a particular dietary regimen, called the "alkalizing diet" or "alkaline diet." The alkalizing or alkaline diet starts from the assumption that the majority of diseases that are capable of affecting our bodies are caused by a real alteration in our pH, which would tend to veer excessively in the direction of acidity.

As the main cause of excessive acidity, the intake of foods with a particularly acidifying action is indicated. An imbalance in the diet followed toward foods with an acidifying action could lead to the onset of cardiovascular disease or chronic inflammatory diseases and more or less serious ailments, from the common cold to cancer. The functioning of our body is based on the delicate acid/base ratio. If this balance is lost and if the environment in which

3

our cells live becomes very acidic, this acidity will penetrate into the cells altering the pH of the nucleus and creating the conditions for those incurable phenomena that are commonly called "cell degeneration diseases." The formation of acids in the body is due in part to the destruction of now-degraded cells, the elimination of which is essential, but which in the long run leads to the formation of ammonia and uric acids, and in part to the choice of foods to bring to our tables.

The determination of the acidity or basicity of a food is made as a result of the analysis of the residual ash remaining following its digestion. These ashes consist predominantly of acidic minerals or basic minerals, and based on this they determine the characteristic associated with the food in question with regard to pH.

It is important to note that there are foods that are at first sight acidic, but are actually capable of causing the body to form useful basic substances. This is, for example, the case with some citrus fruits, among which we find lemons and grapefruits, whose acids are transformed into alkaline (basic) carbohydrates that are useful to the body. This is a process that occurs normally in healthy people, but may not be completely accomplished, due to stress and digestive difficulties, at a time when a person is particularly tired and lacks the energy needed to carry out proper digestion. Stress, as anticipated just above, can be counted among the causes of acidification of the body. Other factors can be added to it, such as smoking, drug intake, sedentary lifestyle, dehydration and consumption of alcoholic beverages. To understand the condition of one's body on the basis of pH, it is necessary to equip oneself with litmus paper, which can be used to assess the level of acidity in urine.

HOW TO RECOGNIZE ACIDIFYING FOODS VS. ALKALIZING FOODS?

Alkaline minerals including sodium, potassium, calcium, and magnesium are likely to be alkalizing to the body if a food has a high concentration of them. Grapes are regarded to be one of the most alkalizing foods. In order to re-balance and purify the body, detoxification diets often use it as a foundation. Some examples of alkalizing foods include spinach and celery as well as dried figs and cucumbers, bean sprouts and lettuce. Ginger, chili peppers, curry, sage, rosemary, fennel seeds, and cumin seeds are all alkalizing seasonings. Quinoa, millet, and amaranth are alkalizing grains (or cereal-like grains).

Acidifying foods include fermented, refined, microwaved, or otherwise highly processed foods that contain sugar and yeast. Grain products are considered acidifying by most nutritionists. Wheat, barley, spelt, oats, rice and rye, as well as their derivatives, such as pasta and bread, are included. Chickpeas, white beans, and lentils are among the legumes that are thought to be acidifying. Acidifying foods include sugar, honey, shrimp, cod, salmon, pork, lamb, cattle, and turkey.

Please note: the alkaline or alkalizing diet does not require one to eliminate acidifying foods from one's diet, but to go in search of balance so that we can avoid excessive acid formation within our bodies. For example, realizing that you

3

are predominantly consuming acidifying foods, you might try to include some alkalizing foods in your diet.

BENEFITS OF THE ALKALINE DIET

Choosing instead to put foods with alkaline power on the table would be a powerful tool we have in our hands to prevent and fight some diseases, including cancer. However, this is a controversial and much debated diet as not all the medical community is convinced of the basis on which the alkaline food theory is based. It must be said, however, that many people who have experimented with this style of eating are actually convinced that it is a useful tool for enjoying good health and can also help increase one's energy intake. But what would be the benefits of this diet? The advantages of following an alkaline diet would be mainly six:

- **Lose weight:** This sort of diet, which focuses on plant-based meals while eliminating animal fats, may aid in weight reduction.

- **Improve health:** those who follow this diet are convinced that it can be especially helpful in the prevention and treatment of inflammation, arthritis and cancer.

- **Have more energy:** thanks to a diet rich in vitamins and minerals, one has the opportunity to see one's energy increase in a short time to benefit the various activities one performs every day.

- **Eliminate hunger pangs:** the alkaline diet allows you to constantly fill up on sugar and fructose. This avoids the sudden hunger pangs that tempt us at certain times of the day and direct us toward the consumption of hydrogenated fats contained in tempting and appetizing snacks that are certainly not the allies of a healthy diet;

- **Managing mood swings:** the continuous intake of sugar in the body stimulates the production of serotonin, the feel-good hormone. As a result, those who follow an alkaline diet will be better able to manage their irritability and sleep better;

- **Improving skin condition:** constant consumption of fruits, vegetables and seeds provides valuable vitamins and minerals. They improve the skin by making it younger, firmer, more elastic and moisturized.

Those who want to experience the benefits for themselves can try following the alkaline diet for 7 days.

ALKALINE DIET: 7-DAYS MEAL PLAN

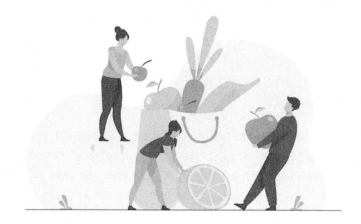

What the alkaline diet allows us to eat are mainly plant-based foods (although not all of them are actually alkalizing, one example for all being wheat and other grains considered acidic). Crucially, it is important to know that we do not have to eliminate acidic foods from our diet altogether, but that the right daily proportion should be to introduce 80 percent alkaline foods and 20 percent acidic foods. We present an example of a weekly alkaline diet menu as a guide only. You can ask an expert to draw up one designed and calibrated to your specific needs.

MONDAY.

- Breakfast: as soon as you wake up, a cup of lukewarm water and lemon. Then a fruit and/or vegetable extract

- Lunch: millet with seasonal vegetables and an apple

- Dinner: Grilled or baked fish seasoned with oil and lemon raw with vegetables

- Snacks: fresh or dried fruit

TUESDAY

- Breakfast: water and lemon and fresh fruit salad
- Lunch: amaranth flan with vegetables
- Dinner: legume soup with raw extra virgin olive oil with a side of vegetables
- Snacks: fruit and vegetable centrifugate or extract

WEDNESDAY

- Breakfast: water and lemon and then fruit or vegetable extract or centrifuge
- Lunch: a quinoa salad with vegetables and dressed with extra virgin olive oil.
- Dinner: tofu with seasonal vegetables
- Snacks: raw vegetables to munch on or fruit

THURSDAY

- Breakfast: water and lemon, fresh seasonal fruit
- Lunch: vegetable and legume soup with croutons
- Dinner: vegetable burger with vegetables
- Snacks: fresh or dried fruit or green tea

FRIDAY

- Breakfast: water and lemon, juice or fruit and vegetable extract

- Lunch: risotto with asparagus or other seasonal vegetables and mixed salad

- Dinner: salmon with potatoes

- Snacks: orange juice or fresh fruit

SATURDAY

- Breakfast: water and lemon, seasonal fruit

- Lunch: whole grain cupcake with vegetables

- Dinner: chickpea hummus with vegetables and whole grain bread

- Snacks: green tea, infusions, fresh or dried fruit

SUNDAY

- Breakfast: water and lemon, fruit salad or extract

- Lunch: big salad with seasonal mixed vegetables, avocado and oil seeds

- Dinner: legume meatballs with a side of vegetables

- Snacks: fresh or dried fruit

CHAPTER 3

ANTI-INFLAMMATORY GUIDE

Inflammation is a chronic illness that may affect everyone and is linked to accelerated aging and a variety of other disorders. To combat it, an anti-inflammatory diet, a genuine health ally, might be beneficial.

Inflammation is a combination of mechanisms by which the body responds to the activity of harmful agents such as bacteria or viruses, as well as external or internal damage. Inflammation often fades after a few days, following the repair of injured tissues and the body's preparedness for full recovery. However, the inflammation may become chronic, subjecting the person to constant variations in severity and duration. It swings between periods when the pain is mild or practically undetectable and times when even the most basic actions become difficult.

Consider the anguish of people who must live with gastritis or arthritis, both of which are typical signs of chronic inflammation, as are Crohn's disease or ulcerative colitis in the intestines. In these circumstances, nutrition, in addition to the advise of the doctor, who will prescribe the appropriate therapy for each of these conditions, may play an important role. There are foods with significant anti-

3

inflammatory characteristics that should be included in one's diet and those that should be avoided. The quantity of calories we consume each day might also aggravate inflammation, particularly when energy intake does not justify its use. Consuming more than we need is never a smart idea.

WHAT IS INFLAMMATION?

Inflammation is a condition that affects all of us occasionally or chronically and is associated with many very common ailments and premature aging. Inflammation consists of a reaction of the body to the action of harmful agents, such as viruses and bacteria, characterized by a set of natural and innate inflammatory processes that the body sets in motion to cope with the infectious, viral, bacterial, traumatic, or toxic event. Under normal conditions inflammation resolves spontaneously after a few days, it can happen, however, that inflammation becomes chronic systemic an insidious and silent mechanism that is defined as *"the set of cellular processes underlying the onset of major chronic degenerative diseases."*

MAIN CAUSES OF INFLAMMATION

The main causes of chronic systemic inflammation are incorrect lifestyles characterized mainly by:

● Unbalanced and often high-calorie diets (i.e., characterized by excessive daily caloric intake) and rich in simple sugars, refined flours, gluten, animal proteins, saturated fats and omega-6.

- Low physical activity and excessively sedentary living

- Pollution

- Psycho-emotional stress over a prolonged period of time

- Abuse of medications

- Alteration of physiological sleep-wake rhythms.

A wrong lifestyle can lead to an alteration of our gut, that is, the organ recognized as our second brain, such that it causes a condition of chronic systemic inflammation. In fact, the gut is responsible for so many sophisticated and fundamental mechanisms of our body such as nutrient absorption and elimination of potentially harmful molecules. In addition, 80% of our immune system and the famous gut microbiome reside in the body.

The gut microbiome is mainly located in the colon and is like a large ecosystem consisting of thousands of microorganisms in a naturally well-structured but extremely fragile and easily altered balance. When the microbiome is altered, conditions are created for the proliferation of pathogens responsible for occasional but also chronic diseases or inflammatory states. An altered microbiome can cause the malabsorption of essential elements (such as vitamin B12, vitamin D, magnesium, iron, etc.) causing a relative organic deficiency, but also the reabsorption of exotoxins and toxic substances and the passage of pro-inflammatory molecules including the infamous free radicals.

THE PRINCIPLE BEHIND THE ANTI-INFLAMMATORY DIET

The anti-inflammatory diet starts with lowering the number of calories we consume via food. Calorie restriction improves inflammation reduction by decreasing the manufacture of pro-inflammatory cytokines. Cytokines are chemicals generated by our bodies that are critical for the development and efficient operation of the immune system. However, if they are created in excess, our bodies may develop inflammatory or autoimmune illnesses.

Calorie restriction in no way means malnutrition, but only a change in the amount of calories normally introduced into our bodies. Taking as reference the intake levels of various nutrients and the recommended calories according to gender and age, it will be enough to reduce calorie consumption by 25 to 30 percent, and vary the sources from which they are obtained. If well applied, calorie reduction:

- Lowers cholesterol and triglyceride levels;

- Increases HDL;

- Enhances telomerase activity, extending cell life;

- Reduces inflammation;

- Combats oxidative stress;

- Counteracts neuro-degenerative diseases;

- Slows down skin aging;

- Stimulates autophagy, a process that renews and keeps tissues and cells clean, promoting the consumption of our reserves. Autophagy is a fundamental process for our cells, and today it is also the subject of some studies for its possible effects on cancer and Alzheimer's.

- Last but not least, calorie restriction also plays an important role in cardiovascular and cerebrovascular aging processes, and combined with regular physical activity increases life expectancy by 5-10 years.

FOODS TO EAT

Food has always been a faithful ally of any therapy. It is safe to say that health is first and foremost won at the table, enriching it with foods that are useful to our bodies for their beneficial properties. Some foods with anti-inflammatory properties are:

- Cereals;

- Whole grain foods;

- Fruits and vegetables; these are also very rich in antioxidants, and have a real protective function of our body against both inflammatory processes and the damage produced by oxidative stress;

- Foods rich in Omega3, an essential source of fatty acids for our body, which alone cannot synthesize them.

4

Here, then, is the importance of introducing them through the diet, either by increasing consumption of fresh fish or through natural supplementation, such as with Krill oil;

- Spices: turmeric, thanks to its active ingredient curcumin, and ginger are potent anti-inflammatories.

FOODS TO AVOID

The first foods to avoid are all types of fats, both saturated and hydrogenated, but also refined flours, excessive consumption of carbohydrates, sugars, dairy products and sausages, red meat and alcohol.

These foods, in fact, promote inflammation, partly because of their ability to lead to the formation of pro-inflammatory toxins and to alter intestinal flora. Inflammatory processes in the intestinal tract are thus promoted. In short, if we think of chronic inflammation as a fire raging inside our bodies, the anti-inflammatory diet is like a canadair that helps us put it out more quickly and effectively!

THE 10 GOLDEN RULES

Going more specific, the foods and preparations that can worsen the state of inflammation and therefore should be avoided could be encapsulated in 10 cornerstones.

1. Fried foods are banned in totality, regardless of the foods and ingredients used.

2. All high-temperature cooking is discouraged; so, for example, if you are on an anti-inflammatory diet, avoid grilling.

3. Minus the allowed glass of red wine per day, spirits are enemies.

4. Excess red meat-small amounts are helpful in providing protein, iron, zinc, selenium, which are needed to optimize healthy and protective inflammatory response-can worsen inflammatory states.

5. No to all foods high in free radicals and saturated fats, such as industrially packaged foods.

6. Important is to reduce consumption of whole cow's milk and its fatty by-products, especially aged cheeses.

7. Control excess refined sugar; better to always prefer whole cane sugar or raw honey.

8. Never overdo salt - if you can, reduce it to the bare minimum.

9. Also decrease consumption of foods with gluten, preferring others that are gluten-free, such as, for example, rice, buckwheat, and quinoa.

10. Avoid eating to the point of maximum fullness.

EXAMPLE MEAL PLAN

After listing inflammatory and anti-inflammatory foods, it is undoubtedly easier to make an example menu based on anti-inflammatory foods.

BREAKFAST

- Green tea or freshly squeezed orange juice (alternatively, another pure fruit juice without added sugar and other additives) or barley;

- One seasonal fruit;

- Half a cup of whole grain cereal or oats (avoid refined grains found in sweets).

LUNCH

- Brown risotto with curry;

- Mixed vegetables dressed with a drizzle of olive oil;

- Greek yogurt with a cup of raspberries and chopped walnuts;

- Water.

SNACK (CHOOSE ONE OR MORE OF THE FOLLOWING)

- Dried fruit or oil seeds such as sunflower or pumpkin seeds; Alternatively, mix of dried fruit and oil seeds;

- Seasonal fruits;

- White yogurt with live milk enzymes;

- Two squares of dark chocolate.

DINNER

- Grilled salmon on a bed of mixed vegetables dressed with a drizzle of olive oil;

- One glass of red wine;

- For dessert, dark chocolate (preferably at least 80 percent);

- Water.

THE PLANT-BASED LIFESTYLE

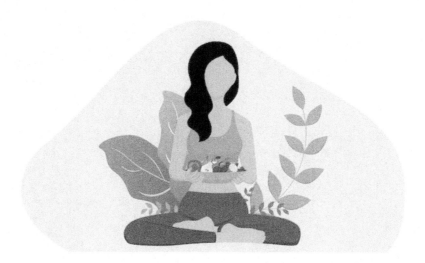

One of the latest food trends is the Plant-Based Diet: but what is it? First of all, to call it a trend, precisely, is very reductive: sure, there are several celebrities who claim to apply the principles of plant-based thinking, but it is much more than a fad.

The plant-based diet is a true approach to life, starting with food: respect for one's own health and body, first and foremost, which is reflected in respect for all forms of life and for the Planet in general. The name itself says a lot "plant-based" means, literally translated, plant-based, thus a predominantly plant-based diet, but not only that. In fact, it is not just about consuming plants but about taking in natural foods: not industrially processed, unprocessed, not derived from resource and animal exploitation, preferably zero miles.

Ethical considerations are combined with a strong health-consciousness: it's best if the food is cruelty-free, and it must be fresh, healthy, balanced, light, and full of essential nutrients. It's a plant-based diet, but it's not vegan or vegetarian. It focuses more on the quality and healthiness of the food than on its "moral" value, but it pays a lot of attention to sustainability.

PLANT BASED VS. VEGAN DIET

The vegan diet involves a diet totally based on plant-based foods: nothing animal-derived is allowed, neither directly nor indirectly, nor any other products-clothing or accessories-that involve the exploitation of animals. No eggs or milk or honey or leather, for that matter, and not only that: in its strictest acceptances, veganism does not even include the use of yeasts, since the bacteria that make them up are unquestionably living beings.

A vegan diet can be balanced, if the person leading it knows well the foods and their combinations, the supplements needed and the reaction of one's physique to the lack of certain foods. In contrast, the Plant-Based diet is on the one hand more relaxed, on the other hand more stringent.

More relaxed because it is plant-based, but not exclusively plant-based: animal products are allowed in moderate amounts, but under one condition, namely the excellent quality of the food itself and its certified provenance. For example, eggs can be consumed occasionally but only if they are very fresh, possibly zero-mile, from free-range farms where hens are not exploited but can live in the open air without constraint.

It is also a philosophy that is somewhat more stringent than veganism for this very reason: as long as it is 100 percent plant-based, the vegan also consumes heavily processed foods, such as industrial chips. In contrast, those who follow the plant-based diet would never allow highly refined foods of this kind.

PLANT-BASED DIETARY APPROACH

Great attention to the quality and nutritional values of foods: no to refined sugars and hydrogenated fats, for example, no to synthetic dyes and sweeteners, no to anything that Mother Nature could not produce spontaneously. But what can you eat, then, if you undertake the plant-based diet?

Green light to whole grains and whole-grain flours, extra virgin olive oil, seasonal fruits and vegetables-these foods are the basis of every meal. Sweets can be eaten only if homemade and with controlled, simple and unrefined raw materials, preferably plant-based-for example, substituting soy or rice drinks for milk, and eggs for other natural thickeners such as flaxseed, psyllium husks or simple ripe banana. Yes to dried fruits and seeds.

Meat and fish? Small amounts of these can be consumed sporadically, as long as they adhere to the main rule of natural and controlled sourcing.

A big NO to everything that is ready-made and processed: ready-made sauces, chips, cookies, snacks of various kinds, sugary cereals, creamy spreads, snacks and many other foods that are known to be very unhealthy. Junk food and fast food are, therefore, absolutely banned!

HEALTH BENEFITS

Eating mainly fresh, seasonal fruits and vegetables, cooked simply without overdoing the seasonings, combined with unrefined grains and flours, few sugars, lots of water: sounds like the perfect health recipe. Obviously it needs to be studied with a professional but, if well structured and planned, it is a diet that can give great benefits in terms of weight loss, cardiovascular health, diabetes-related problems, hypertension and inflammation.

In fact, you get your fill of micronutrients: minerals, such as calcium, iron, magnesium, potassium and zinc, and vitamins such as A, C, E and folic acid, but also plant sterols, which fight cholesterol, and fiber, which helps gut health. We also find some really portentous antioxidants in plants, such as polyphenols, anthocyanins and carotenoids, for example the lycopene contained in tomatoes, which are valuable for their natural anti-inflammatory properties.

ECO-SUSTAINABILITY AND FOOD AWARENESS

To embark on this path, one must be a mindful consumer: if you are used to shopping by putting only special offers and refined foods loaded with fat and sugar in your cart... it will be difficult to take this step, but not impossible. You have to learn to read product labels, both as ingredients and as the origin and processing of the products. Only by really knowing what you put on the table-such as provenance and nutritional values-can you understand whether it is suitable for this dietary regimen.

And not only that: consuming fresh foods means following seasonality. In October you eat pumpkin, in July you eat watermelon, it cannot be otherwise: expecting to eat strawberries in December and chestnuts in June creates the need to force nature's hand with intensive greenhouse cultivation and processing to preserve foods beyond the correct season. This focus on following nature's rhythm, avoiding industrial forcing, is good for the environment, although plant-based is more about health than the purely ethical choice of veganism.

PLANT-BASED MEAL PLAN EXAMPLE

Wanting to try to sketch a daily menu of the plant diet for weight loss, one can follow this scheme:

- Breakfast: fresh fruit in addition 2 whole wheat cookies and some unsweetened tea;

- Lunch: vegetables of your choice (preferably raw) in addition 50-80 g whole wheat pasta with cherry tomatoes and boiled chickpeas;

- Dinner: again vegetables of your choice (preferably raw) with in addition sea bass or a sea bream and fruit.

- Snacks can be added to this pattern either in the morning or in the afternoon with fresh or dried fruit.

This is an example of a plant-based diet menu.Of course, we repeat it every time we describe any kind of diet regimen, the advice is always to consult a professional who can give you a personalized diet plan and the right advice to avoid health risks.

CHAPTER 5

MEET DR. SEBI

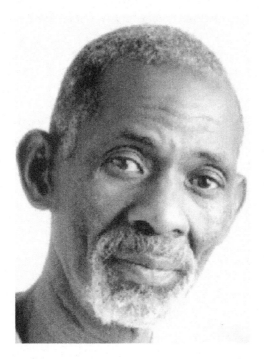

Throughout history, great men have attempted to alleviate mankind's suffering by curing the body and treating maladies that Western medicine thought incurable. Since Wilhelm Reich discovered orgone energy and constructed an orgone-storage device that helped treat hundreds of individuals of a variety of illnesses, we've gone from Royal Rife to Rife.

In both cases, the existing medical establishment and its trillions of dollars in annual earnings from cancer therapies were endangered by these two great men's discoveries. During the time he was being sued, Royal Rife's discoveries and the frequency healing machine were utterly destroyed, even though he won the case. A man named Wilhelm Reich was also sued and imprisoned, but he suddenly died there. Furthermore, all of his orgone energy research was also destroyed. As it turns out, the individual to whom this chapter is devoted also met with a tragic end.

There were accusations that Dr. Sebi had been poisoned while in prison because of his holistic healing methods. He was derided for developing a natural cure for HIV/AIDS, cancer, and other maladies. People like Michael Jackson and Steven Seagal and Eddie Murphy and John Travolta were healed by him. Nipsey Hussle and Lisa Lopes, two of these celebrities, were so grateful for Dr. Sebi's counsel and healing that they wanted to demonstrate their thanks by promoting his healing methods and treatments.

Nipsey Hussle announced that she will fund and produce a documentary about Dr. Sebi. However, before the documentary could be completed, Nipsey Hussle was found dead, having been shot many times. Lisa Lopes was working on a documentary about Dr. Sebi's life and spiritual journey, in which he played an important role. Unfortunately, she died tragically in a vehicle accident not long after meeting him. But who was this mysterious figure known as Dr. Sebi? And what was it about his therapeutic methods and practices that made them so effective in curing so many people?

THE BIRTH OF A MYTH

Alfredo Darrington Bowman, better known as Dr. Sebi, was born in a small Honduran hamlet in 1933. Alfredo spent his early years as a machinist aboard a cargo ship, traveling all over the world. He did not live a healthy lifestyle and ate excessively, thus he quickly gained weight. By the age of 35, he was suffering from major health issues, including asthma, diabetes, impotence, eyesight problems, and obesity.

He traveled to the United States in search of relief from modern Western medicine, but soon learned that conventional medical treatment had little effect on him. As his condition worsened, he started to explore for other options. During his travels, he heard about a man who used herbs and natural medicine to practice various old healing procedures. So he traveled to Mexico to visit Alfredo Cortez, a herbalist. He was dying, according to the Mexican healer, but he also knew how to help him.

First, he told him to fast for 90 days, eating nothing and drinking only water. During this time, the herbalist gave him various combinations of natural herbs and juice on occasion. Then she told him to go on a vegetarian diet and not to drink any milk or meat. At the end of the process, the Mexican herbalist had entirely healed Alfredo Bowman of all medical ailments. Alfredo was so motivated by this miraculous turnaround that he went on to become Dr. Sebi and further his understanding of natural herbal therapy, fasting, and the vegan alkaline diet.

DR. SEBI'S DIET

Dr. Sebi began cataloging many herbs, plants, and fungus in the years that followed. Then he experimented on his own body, consuming numerous combinations of treatments and fasting regimens. He studied numerous indigenous healing practices from Africa, Central America, and the Caribbean and was fully self-taught. This formerly enormous and helpless guy, who suffered from asthma, diabetes, and visual difficulties, would achieve peak health and father approximately twenty children by the end of his life. His research, fasting, and plant cataloguing eventually led him to establish his alkaline healing known as "African bio-electric cellular food treatment."

Dr. Sebi felt that diseases are caused by the production of mucus within our bodies' various cells. Because mucus stops oxygen from reaching the cells, they degrade. Excess mucus accumulation, for example, in the lungs causes pneumonia, whereas excess mucus in the pancreas causes diabetes. According to him, illnesses can only exist in acidic surroundings. As a result, he used his alkaline plant-based diet, as well as numerous plants, to produce an alkaline condition in the body and so eradicate ailments. Only natural alkaline fruits, cereals, veggies, nuts, and legumes were consumed.

Traditional therapeutic plants such as turmeric, burdock root, linden flower, dandelion root, and others were used in the herbal mixtures he made. He also employed various types of sea moss, which boosts the immune system and provides vitality. Dr. Sebi's alkaline diet, fasting protocol, and herbal medicines were designed to cleanse the body's

5

cells at the cellular and intracellular levels, as well as detoxify and recharge the immune system. The benefits of the various herbs utilized by Dr. Sebi, as well as the benefits of adopting a vegan diet and intermittent fasting, have long been backed by science.

Drinking plenty of spring water was another important part of Dr. Sebi's diet. Because the human body is 70% water, this is important for the alkaline diet to work. Because many of the herbs used to detoxify the body are diuretics and increase urine, regular hydration with spring water is essential.

THE WESTERN COMPARISON

After successfully healing and assisting hundreds of people in Honduras, Dr. Sebi moved to the United States and established his own business selling herbal treatments and treating individuals. He also treated numerous Americans and swiftly rose to prominence in the country. With the proceeds from his labor, he founded the Usha healing community in Honduras, which he named after his eldest daughter Usha Bowman.

The Usha community swiftly became a world-renowned center for natural medicine, with individuals traveling thousands of miles to receive treatment. The village was magnificently set in nature, with natural therapeutic hot springs, and therapies included steam baths and hot spring spas.

Dr. Sebi's renown grew too high in the United States, and the FDA sued him in 1988 for practicing without a license and fraudulent advertising. While it was obvious that Dr. Sebi lacked a license and a medical degree, was this truly misleading advertising? He claimed in his commercials that he could heal cancer, leukemia, lupus, herpes, AIDS, and a variety of other diseases, some of which were thought to be incurable.

Dr. Sebi filed a Supreme Court challenge against the New York Attorney General, and the judge ordered Sebi to submit a witness for each of the ailments he claimed to have healed. Furthermore, each witness was required to bring a certificate verified by an independent doctor demonstrating that he had the specific ailment, as well as another document certified by a different doctor proving that the witness was now cured of that illness. The judge, the attorney general, and everyone who had been following the case were taken aback when 77 witnesses appeared in court with Dr. Sebi, carrying the necessary paperwork confirming healing. Despite being questioned for hours and having his herbal treatments analyzed by various laboratories, Dr. Sebi was eventually declared not guilty.

SUSPICIOUS FACTS

The process backfired and increased his popularity. He also began working with a number of superstars, including Michael Jackson, Steven Segal, Eddie Murphy, John Travolta, Magic Johnson, and others. Dr. Sebi's African Bio-Electric Food Therapy assisted Michael Jackson in overcoming a morphine and painkiller addiction. He also used herbs to treat Steven Segal's five-year severe headache.

More lawsuits would follow, but Dr. Sebi's fame grew nevertheless. The FDA was powerless to stop him since an increasing number of people believed his claims and claimed to have been cured. Lisa (Left Eye) Lopes, lead singer of TLC, was one of several patients who expressed gratitude to Dr. Sebi. He assisted her in overcoming her addictions to alcohol, cigarettes, and despair. Lisa's life was drastically revolutionized as a result, and she frequently stated that Dr. Sebi had opened her eyes. Lisa intended to repay him by disseminating knowledge about him and his healing techniques, as well as sharing her own change. So she told MTV about her experience at Usha Village.

Lisa later began work on a documentary on his life, in which Dr. Sebi and the Usha village played an important role. She frequently visited the Honduran community of Usha until she unfortunately perished in a car accident one day after meeting with Dr. Sebi. Many people feel Lisa Lopez's death was not an accident and that it was necessary to put an end to her quest to popularize Dr. Sebi and his holistic healing practices.

Nipsey Hussle, the famous rapper, was another thankful patient of Dr. Sebi. Dr. Sebi was so appreciative that after his death, he wanted to support the making of an entire documentary about him and his healing procedures. Nipsey Hussle was fatally shot shortly after beginning work on the documentary. Many others believe he was murdered in order to raise awareness of Dr. Sebi's holistic treatment practices around the world. The death of a high-profile celebrity linked to Dr. Sebi has heightened suspicions.

THE END OF DR. SEBI

Attacks against Dr. Sebi became more severe, and the attorney general's office even dispatched undercover operatives to pose as patients in need of healing in order to uncover any anomalies in Dr. Sebi's procedures. Dr. Sebi was arrested at the airport on money laundering accusations on May 28, 2016, because he was carrying $37,000 in cash. Despite the fact that he, his friends, family, and patients all refuted the money laundering claims, Sebi was imprisoned.

Dr. Sebi's company was generating a lot of money selling healing medicines at the time, and Sebi himself was making a lot of money from personal healing sessions with all types of people, including celebrities. So all that was required to exonerate Dr. Sebi was a certificate from his company proving the source of the funds. His family called the company several times to collect the necessary documentation; however, no one from the corporation returned their calls or attempted to assist Dr. Sebi in any way.

When a high-profile person, such as Dr. Sebi, is arrested on allegations such as money laundering, he should be given a court date for a hearing as soon as possible, as well as a bond amount that he can pay to remain out of detention until his trial. Dr. Sebi received neither because there was no court date scheduled and no bail was granted. He was regarded as if he were a murderer rather than a healer. All he could do was wait in the dreadful surroundings of the prison.

After a few months, Dr. Sebi informed his daughter that they were attempting to poison him with the food provided to him in prison. Even though he was 82 years old, everyone knew he was in good health because he demonstrated it all the time. However, authorities stated in August 2016 that Dr. Sebi died in prison after contracting pneumonia. Shortly after his death, the firm he built from scratch, the same company that did nothing to assist him, registered his name and seized his inheritance.

Many people, including Dr. Sebi's first wife and eldest daughter, stated that the treatments sold by his company were not the original therapeutic formula. Consumers have also stated that the recipe was changed as a result of several of them having horrible responses and adverse effects. Dr. Sebi's huge danger to the multibillion-dollar medical business, which relies on the continuance of diseases and therapies through chemical and unnatural means, was over. They eventually succeeded in permanently silenced Dr. Sebi and dispersed his legacy.

His death was not even mentioned in the main publications. How is this possible, given that Dr. Sebi demonstrated in court that he could naturally treat cancer, leukemia, lupus, herpes, aids, and a variety of other diseases, with over 70 witnesses to back him up? Why hasn't this outstanding man received more attention?

Who would pay thousands and thousands of dollars for chemotherapy and synthetic medications if it was known that we could heal cancer with fasting, a vegetarian diet, and alkaline herbal remedies? The pharmaceutical business alone is worth $1.27 trillion, and it is rising at a rapid pace. People take drugs to treat headaches, insomnia, sadness, and, lastly, diseases and maladies. Imagine how successful the medical industry would be if everyone adopted Dr. Sebi's ways instead of medicine.

CHAPTER 6

THE POWER OF FASTING

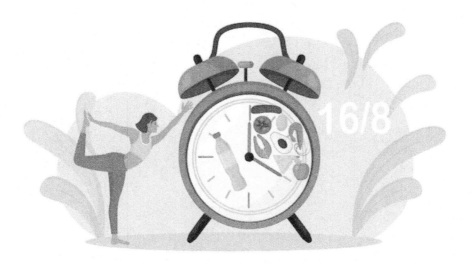

Fasting is an ancient practice, carried out historically for reasons related to religion. More recently, it has attracted the attention of researchers who realized how cutting calories helped people live fitter and longer. This was the starting point for a series of studies on fasting, understood precisely as a reduction (sometimes very drastic) in energy intake during the day.

Fasting has numerous health benefits and has assisted people in gaining better control of their health and reversing symptoms of a variety of conditions. However, it has grown in favor as a rapid technique to lose weight, however the effects frequently result in the dreaded yoyo effect. This chapter will discuss the myths surrounding fasting to lose weight, how to actually harness the power of fasting to permanently lose weight, and which types of fasting are most beneficial for obtaining long-term weight reduction outcomes.

To lose weight, we are advised that we must generate a calorie deficit, which means that we must burn more calories than we consume each day. Most experts and nutritionists will advise you to increase your physical activity and eliminate meals with high calorie intake but few nutritional advantages, commonly known as empty calories. However, many people resort to procedures that appear to be quick cures, such as fasting, in order to lose weight quickly. Although it seems to be a simple technique to lose weight rapidly, there are numerous myths and misconceptions that may cause you to gain weight in the long run.

WHAT IS THE FASTING DIET?

The fasting diet, also known as the "mimic fasting" diet, involves the controlled intake of protein (11-14 percent), carbohydrates (42-43 percent) and fat (46 percent), for an overall calorie reduction of between 34 and 54 percent from canonical intake. Under this label, two types of diets fall. The 5:2 diet stipulates that for five days a week, one can eat taking in all foods, without exception. The period must be interspersed with two days (non-consecutive with each other) in which the energy intake must be no more than a quarter of the usual one: that is, between 500 and 600 kilocalories (200-250 at breakfast and 300-350 at dinner). An intermittent fasting diet is also referred to when food intake is concentrated in a period of between 6 and 8 hours (16/8 pattern). Even the smallest snack is avoided before the start of the day and after the final meal, in order to acclimatize the body to living and "working" under conditions of reduced fullness. By doing so, energy is also saved at the end of the day, which happens to individuals who are accustomed to eating supper late, leaving no opportunity to expend the collected energy before going to bed.

THE BENEFITS OF INTERMITTENT FASTING

The benefits of calorie restriction have been known for decades and have been summarized by Rafael de Cabo (Laboratory of Translational Gerontology, National Institute of Aging, Baltimore) and Mark Mattson (Department of Neuroscience, Johns Hopkins University) in the review published in one of the world's leading medical journals. "Intermittent eating is a choice that can be part of a healthy lifestyle," said Mattson himself, a follower of the intermittent fasting diet for 20 years. The most compelling data involves the preservation of appropriate cell health at the organ level. Depleting glucose stores and depending on fat as an energy source allows the process to take place. According to Mattson, this improves "blood glucose management, reduces inflammatory response, and increases resilience to stress." Based on four investigations in both animal models and humans, the compilation discovered that "intermittent fasting also decreased blood pressure, blood lipid levels, and resting heart rate." Less robust, but still present in the literature, is evidence documenting an impact on obesity and the risk of getting diabetes.

The paper also echoes the findings of several preliminary epidemiological studies from the conclusions of which suggest that intermittent fasting--replicating the same mechanism mentioned above--may also promote the maintenance of brain health and thus have a potential preventive role against diseases such as stroke, Alzheimer's and Parkinson's. Although much research is still needed before demonstrating the effects of intermittent fasting on learning and memory, according to Mattson, it cannot be ruled out that "in the future, the intermittent fasting diet may become one of the possibilities for preventing or at least delaying the onset of a neurodegenerative process."

There are several aspects to consider, however, before considering adopting such an eating regimen. Especially in the beginning, following a drastic change in one's lifestyle habits, a person may find it difficult to cope with the feelings of hunger and irritability that can occur in the first few weeks. For this reason, as always when dieting (in this case, slimming is not the most relevant benefit), it is essential to be followed by an experienced specialist. This is also because, although it is not a true fast, such a dietary regimen is not suitable for everyone and is not recommended, for example, for children, growing children, pregnant women, the elderly, and people struggling with a chronic illness. And it should in any case be followed for a limited period of time.

EATING ADVICE DURING FASTING

During fasting, you will optimally consume very few calories, depending on the method you choose. Some even opt for water fasting, which essentially means that during the fasting period you will consume nothing but water. However, this is frequently unhealthy and, in some cases, dangerous.

Many people believe that this provides the greatest calorie deficit because every calorie you expend is not compensated with a calorie consumed. And, because food is not introduced into the body, the body is forced to locate fresh energy stores inside itself. This occurs when the body depletes its fat reserves. However, if the body believes it is in starvation mode due to a lack of calories, it may begin to consume muscle or put undue stress to key organs. This procedure deprives the body not only of calories, but also of minerals and electrolytes that allow important processes to continue operating while fasting.

There are additional health dangers when reintroducing food into the body if fasting is not done under the right supervision of a medical practitioner or expert. Because of the body's perceived hunger, unexpected changes in electrolyte balances and calorie intake can create a re-feeding syndrome, causing extra stress to the internal organs and systems.

WHAT HAPPENS WHEN WE FAST?

In the history of human evolution, for a long time (centuries) food was not available all the time and everywhere as (but not for everyone) it is today. This means that the human body is made to tolerate moments of fasting and alternate them with moments of eating. Scientific studies have shown that those (humans and other animals) who regularly perform moments of fasting live longer, are less likely to develop cancers and maintain their mental faculties better in old age. In fact, fasting triggers stress-response reactions in the body that are beneficial in the long run.

Here is what happens in our bodies when we do not eat: after 8 hours from the start of fasting, the body will have exhausted the supply of glucose (the essential fuel for life) introduced with the last meal, and will begin to produce it using the glycogen stores in the liver. As the fasting continues, the body uses, to produce glucose, the glycogen stores stored in the muscles and later (about 12 hours after the fasting begins) those in the adipose tissue, "burning fat," to be clear. Burning fat is our mirage, and this might make us think of fasting as a single remedy for losing weight.

Beware, however: the chemical reactions involved also produce ketone bodies as metabolic waste, and these in large quantities are toxic to the body. Continuing fasting "to the bitter end" (when fat reserves fall below 7 percent of body weight) causes the body to start using protein to obtain glucose: this is where slimming ends and wasting begins. It is not advisable to do fasts lasting longer than three weeks. Well-organized and prepared fasting leads to

6

the elimination of recently consumed toxins, a decrease in inflammation, and a strengthening of the immune system (which is no longer forced to go into operation at every meal to check the "non-belligerence" of absorbed food particles). In addition, as we know, cancer cells have quite a need for energy: leaving them fasting as well can help slow or prevent their development. These mechanisms of detoxification and elimination of toxins can manifest themselves during fasting in various forms: headaches, diarrhea, skin manifestations, mild widespread pain. All should disappear within 1-2 days.

FASTING VADEMECUM

Given the costs and benefits of fasting, here are some tips for those who want to approach it. Do not do fasts longer than 1-2 days without notifying your doctor or otherwise hearing your doctor's advice. Do not fast if you are diabetic, if you are under 21 years of age or if you have other ongoing medical conditions (if so, ask your doctor). Recommendations:

- Before starting the actual fast, begin body purification with 2 days of only fresh, preferably raw, seasonal fruits and vegetables.

- Drink plenty during the fast, water (preferably water with low fixed residue and pH between 6.4 and 6.9) or even vegetable centrifuges or vegetable broth, to help flush out toxins and maintain the necessary hydration.

- If you feel excessively hungry during fasting, you can exceptionally consume one or two fresh fruits.

- Choose appropriate days for fasting, especially for the first time: avoid days of extreme stress or physically strenuous work. Better to start on a weekend and see how it goes.

- Do the fast for no more than 1-2 days and resume eating fresh raw vegetables and fruits for at least two more days, before resuming a diet that is as light and healthy as possible, so as not to immediately nullify the beneficial effects of fasting.

- It is also possible to repeat the fast, if well tolerated, once a month.

CHAPTER 7

HEALTHY HABITS

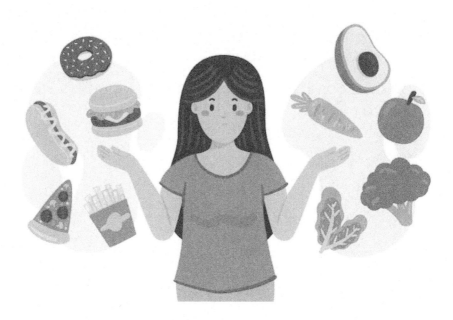

To function properly, our bodies require good eating habits. Thus, a balanced intake of nutrients is essential, including carbs, fats, proteins, minerals, and vitamins. The requirement for these components changes according to age, physiological circumstances (pregnancy, sports, etc.), and the presence of any disorders. Because no one item has all of the required components in the proper amount and balance, our diet must be as diverse as possible. We are familiar with two fundamental approaches to the realm of nutrition:

- Food information: being up-to-date on food and nutrition.

- Nutrition education: acquiring food practices to eat well.

This necessitates a shift in lifestyle. What we eat and how we cook it, the ingredients we use: these are some of the healthy eating habits that might affect our health and body's functioning.

BEST DIETARY PRACTICES

Examining our behaviors allows us to have a deeper knowledge of not just ourselves and our real lifestyle, but also of the food culture of the nation in which we live and the socioeconomic changes that are taking place there.

RESPECT THE 5 MEALS OF THE DAY

Taking at least 5 breaks every day (breakfast, morning snack, lunch, snack, and supper) enhances food absorption, avoids obesity, eases digestion, and helps us to maintain consistent energy levels.

DRINK 2 LITERS OF WATER DAILY

Hydrating the body properly is a healthy technique that allows for better physical and mental performance. Water also has a cleaning and purifying impact, which aids in the removal of impurities from our bodies. In addition to using smartphone applications to encourage higher fluid consumption, you may undertake the following basic practices:Always keep a bottle handy.

- Don't wait until you are thirsty before drinking.

- Between drinks you can introduce infusions of tea or mint.

- Pay attention to weather changes to vary your consumption.

- Drinking sugary, carbonated or alcoholic drinks is not healthy; in fact, it is one of the classic points to avoid. Water is the only real source of hydration for the body.

EAT WHOLE FRUITS ON AN EMPTY STOMACH

Eating water-rich meals like veggies assists you to maintain your body's water balance. Fruit pieces are preferred to fruit beverages, which are high in sugar and low in nutrients.

AVOID HIGHLY PROCESSED FOODS

Highly processed meals, such as sweets, baked goods, and fast foods, are depleted of nutrients and deliver empty calories. The addition of colours, sugars, and preservatives in these meals is another detrimental element impacting health. A favorable attitude about avoiding certain items is to:

- Replace them with natural food such as fruit for snacks.

- Avoiding the purchase of ready-made meals, cakes and various sweets.

CONSUMPTION OF FOODS RICH IN OMEGA 3

Looking for good eating habits? Omega 3 and 6 fatty acids are vital since the body cannot generate them and must obtain them from diet. Omega 6 is abundant in meals, however omega 3 is more difficult to come by.

This imbalance puts you at risk for cardiovascular disease, cancer, and autoimmune illnesses. To compensate for this imbalance, consume omega-3-rich foods such as flaxseed and fatty fish such as sardines, salmon, and mackerel.

REDUCE CONSUMPTION OF MEAT AND DAIRY PRODUCTS

Milk and dairy products in general have high levels of cholesterol and arachidonic acid, which is a precursor to inflammatory mediators and allergic reactions. As a result, it is advised to consume soy milk, which is high in isoflavones, flavonoid chemicals with strong anti-cancer properties.

Isoflavones function similarly to human estrogen in that they ameliorate or avoid menopausal symptoms, especially when used routinely from a young age. Soy products such as beans, tofu, miso, tempeh, and yogurt offer the same advantages.

Meat is also a danger factor for humans, especially when it comes to cardiovascular disease and issues associated with overburdening the organs responsible for eliminating toxins. Antibiotics and hormones may be present in meat.

These are the compounds utilized in intensive animal farms; plant-based feeds such as legumes are a great substitute (chickpeas, lentils, peas, beans, broad beans).

DECREASE SALT INTAKE

A high-salt diet is frequently the cause of hypertension. It is critical to develop the habit of utilizing herbs and spices as salt alternatives, minimize intake of high-sodium canned and ready-made meals, study product labels, and pick those with lower sodium levels. Finally, do not add more salt to a cooked food.

PLANNING A DIETARY PROGRAM

Cells in the body function similarly to biological clocks. This is also true for our biological functioning, which is why eating in a systematic manner is crucial. It is beneficial to design an eating schedule that keeps track of the calories ingested throughout the day and distributes them at each meal. For example, a robust breakfast may be followed by a lighter lunch.

INCREASE FIBER INTAKE

Fiber is beneficial to our bodies because it has a cleansing and detoxifying impact, improves cholesterol levels, avoids constipation, and aids in the maintenance of a healthy weight. Fresh fruits, vegetables, and nuts are excellent sources of fiber and should not be overlooked in our diet.

WRONG DIETARY SOLUTIONS TO AVOID

- Eating out of meals: have small snacks throughout the day.

- Exaggerating with ready-made meals: they are high in fat, sugar and salt.

- Shopping when you are hungry: buy unnecessary products.

- Eating out: exceed quantities and consume caloric foods.

This subject has to be diversified and balanced. As it can aid in the avoidance of pathological illnesses, a correct regimen is associated with health protection and maintenance. Let us not forget that a balanced diet should always be linked with exercise and sports activity in order to support whole body growth and preserve maximum health.

HABITS FOR BETTER LIVING

Who said routine is unhealthy? Routines may really help you live a better life because they provide you with goals to strive towards, which help you stay focused. It is difficult to keep focused with all that you have to do: job, family, and home. It might be tough to reconcile everything. That is why it is beneficial to develop habits that will help us enhance our life and our health. We advocate the following eight healthy behaviors to live a healthier life:

1) Follow a morning routine

The course of our day is determined by how we begin it. We are always more enthusiastic in the morning, yet we frequently rush about, which increases our stress levels. Our advice is to wake up early and enjoy breakfast, to take your time getting ready for the day, and to make a list of things to accomplish during the day to help you create daily objectives.

2) Eating healthy

The cornerstone idea for individuals who desire to live happier and healthier lives is to eat a healthy and balanced diet. It is critical not to skip the three main meals and instead dine out: in fact, one study found that eating uncontrolled can raise the chance of developing diabetes. Furthermore, consuming a variety of fruits and vegetables enhances immunity and lowers the risk of heart disease and cancer.

3) Drink plenty of water

Our bodies are 70% water, which is required not just to hydrate us but also to maintain our body temperature, transport nutrients to cells, and remove waste. Drinking at least 8 glasses of water every day is a good habit to form.

4) Have regular sleep

Sleeping is not only a time for our bodies to relax, but it is also a time for detoxification: while we sleep, a sequence of critical mechanisms in our bodies are engaged, which heal our bodies from the damage done during the day. Our recommendation for healthier living is to sleep at least 8 hours a night and have regular routines, so that you always go to sleep and wake up at the same time, so that the usual "sleep-wake" cycle is not disrupted.

5) Do physical activity

You should exercise for at least 30 minutes every day to boost blood circulation and metabolism. We offer modest ploys to move more when you can't attend a gym class or don't have time to run, such as stretching as soon as you wake up in the morning, parking your car away from your job to walk a bit, or even preferring the stairs to the elevator.

6) Do not smoke

Smoking is bad for your health since it harms your respiratory and cardiovascular systems and is one of the primary causes of cancer. It can induce infertility in both men and women, and it can be much more detrimental to children who are passively exposed to it, as it raises the chance of respiratory and ear infections.

7) Turn off the TV and smartphone

We are compelled to spend up to 8 hours a day, for leisure or job, in front of a bright screen that constantly stimulates our brain activity. To detox, we recommend not turning on your mobile phone as soon as you wake up in the morning, not carrying cell phones or laptops with you at all times to avoid interaction with electromagnetic radiation, and finally, turn off the TV at least an hour before going to bed.

8) Have regular checkups

Prevention is an excellent ally for those who want to live healthy. Few people in America still take regular blood tests or adhere to screening programs. Often, the fear that something might be discovered leads to total disinterest. One should not be alarmist, but our advice is not to underestimate preventive medical checkups.

With a little effort, these 8 good habits can be followed every day. Don't wait until tomorrow to start. Start now!

FOOD HABITS TO DETOX YOUR BODY

Especially after a period of excesses at the table or when we lead an excessively sedentary life, it is essential to detoxify our bodies. This essentially translates into helping the "filter organs" (the technical term is "emunctory organs") through food, that is, those whose function is to eliminate waste products from our bodies, and these are the liver and kidneys. It is therefore necessary to consume detoxifying foods, which help these two organs to perform their function well because, when they are overloaded, the body ends up expelling waste products through the skin or respiratory system i.e., through dermatitis, phlegm, coughs and other respiratory tract infections.

It is probably unnecessary by now to point out that the foods that help the body are mainly fruits and vegetables, but how to choose them? Let's look at it below. Among the most useful foods for detoxifying the body (that is, eliminating toxins) are:

- Artichokes: stimulate liver metabolism and have a protective function towards the liver parenchyma;

- Chicories: contain phosphorus, calcium and vitamin A, are rich in minerals, but poor in heat, good for diuresis and bowel function;

- Apples: help digestion and reduce toxins, contain calcium, iron, potassium and phosphorus, and simplify diuresis;

- Carrots: help both the liver and kidneys, purify the blood, regularize bowel function and are diuretic;

- Milk thistles: protect the liver thanks to detoxifying medicinal substances they contain, so much so that they are also used in cases of fungal poisoning;

- Oranges: are rich in vitamins C, A, E, PP, B1, B2, B5 and B6; they help digestion, liver and intestines;

- Grapefruits: have a positive effect on liver, kidneys, gastric juices (and therefore digestion). They also facilitate intestinal transit, diuresis and absorption of sugars and fats;

- Blueberries: have anti-inflammatory effects and improve circulation;

- Grapes: contain sugars, minerals, vitamins and promote the production of gastric juices.

In addition to being especially careful in choosing detoxifying foods, it is also good to start adopting some eating habits that certainly help our bodies. First of all we need to reduce salt consumption, because the recommended dose is only 6 grams per day per person (which is what is contained in one pizza). Then avoid fatty sauces and replace them with yogurt-based sauces, which is a food that lends a big hand to the bacterial flora.

Also recommended are purifying herbal teas made with artichoke, birch or elderberry. Perhaps substitute them for salty snacks. And to sweeten them, it is best to use honey.

QUICK & EASY HEALTHY RECIPES

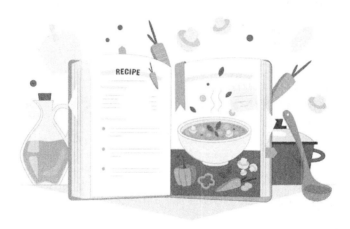

The first rule of gaining and maintaining mental and physical well-being is to eat healthily and in a balanced manner. A healthy diet, in reality, provides great benefits to our immune system and aids in the prevention of bodily problems and chronic diseases. This area has a variety of healthy and appetizing recipes that will help you protect your health without sacrificing the delights of good eating! In addition to describing all of the processes for cooking dishes in detail, our health recipes will teach you about the beneficial characteristics and nutritional values of the goods that nature provides.

BREAKFAST & SNACKS

SPINACH FRITTATA

Time to prepare: 20 minutes

Time to cook: 30 minutes

4 servings

INGREDIENTS

- 8 medium eggs
- 6 tsp black pepper (to taste)
- 12 tsp garlic powder
- 12 tsp dried thyme
- 12 tsp red pepper flakes
- 12 cup parmesan cheese, grated
- 12 medium diced onion (3 oz)
- 1 bag fresh spinach, finely chopped

INSTRUCTIONS

1. Heat the oven to 400°F. Place an ungreased 9-inch ceramic or glass cake pan in the oven to warm along with the oven.

2. In a large mixing bowl, whisk together the eggs, black pepper, garlic powder, dried thyme, and red pepper flakes.

3. Mix in the Parmesan cheese and onion. Then, in batches, mix in the spinach.

4. Remove the hot cake pan from the oven with oven mitts and set it on a trivet. Grease the baking dish lightly.

5. Fill the heated cake pan halfway with the egg and spinach mixture. Use a rubber spatula to smooth the top. It may appear that there is a lot of spinach compared to eggs, but keep in mind that spinach wilts when cooking.

6. Place the pan back in the oven. Bake the frittata for 25 to 30 minutes, or until it has risen up and a toothpick inserted into the center comes out clean.

7. Allow the frittata to cool in the pan for 15 minutes before cutting it into eight triangles and serving.

110kcal | 2g carbohydrate | 10g protein | 7g fat | 3g saturated fat | 273mg sodium | 1g fiber | 1g sugar

BANANA BREAD

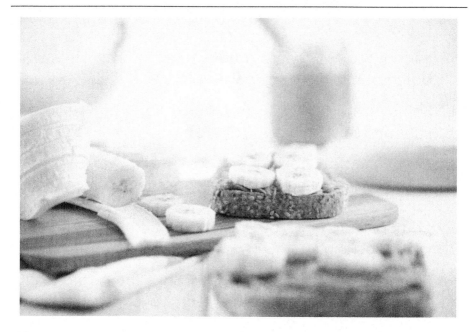

Time to prepare: 15 minutes

Time to cook: 50 minutes

12 slices

INGREDIENTS

- Spray the pan with cooking spray (I use avocado oil spray)
- three huge eggs
- 3 big, ripe bananas, well mashed (1.5 cups)
- 1 tbsp. vanilla extract
- 2 teaspoons honey

- 2 cups almond meal, blanched and finely ground (8 oz)
- * 1 tablespoon cinnamon powder
- 1 tablespoon baking soda

INSTRUCTIONS

1. Heat the oven to 350°F. Line a small baking sheet (8.5 X 4.5 inches) with baking paper strips, allowing an overhang on either side. Spray the lined baking sheet lightly with oil.

2. In a medium-sized mixing bowl, combine the eggs, mashed bananas, vanilla extract, and sweetener.

3. Gradually stir in the almond flour, cinnamon, and baking soda. Blend until completely smooth.

4. Transfer the batter to the prepared baking pan with a rubber spatula. Tap the pan gently on the work surface to disperse the batter evenly.

5. Bake the banana bread for 40 to 50 minutes, or until golden brown and firm and a toothpick inserted into the center comes out dry.

6. Carefully take the banana bread from the baking sheet, using the leftover baking paper as a handle, and place it on a wire rack to cool. Remove the baking paper carefully to let air to flow.

7. Allow the bread to cool entirely on a cooling rack for approximately 2 hours. Serve it cut into 12 pieces.

172kcal | 15g carbohydrate | 6g protein | 11g fat | 1g saturated fat | 147mg sodium | 3g fiber | 8g sugar

EGGS BENEDICT

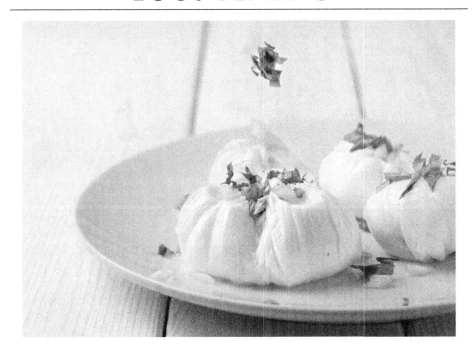

Time to prepare: 30 minutes

Time to cook: 15 minutes

Servings: 2

INGREDIENTS FOR BAKE:

- 3 tbsp unsalted butter, split
- 2 huge eggs, separated
- divided 2 tablespoons coconut flour
- 12 tsp baking powder (divided; gluten-free if needed)

MAKE THE HOLLANDAISE SAUCE AS FOLLOWS:

- 1 big yolk of an egg
- 1 tablespoon water
- 1 teaspoon freshly squeezed lemon juice
- 1 tsp cayenne pepper
- 8 tbsp unsweetened butter

TO PUT TOGETHER:

- two huge eggs
- 2 pieces Canadian bacon

INSTRUCTIONS

Make the bread:

1. Melt 1 tablespoon butter in a small microwave-safe bowl (mine measures 3 inches at the bottom and 3.5 inches at the top).

2. Allow it cool somewhat before adding one egg, 1 tablespoon coconut flour, and 14 teaspoon baking powder. Stir the mixture slowly until it is smooth.

3. Microwave the mixture for 90 seconds at high power. When removing from the microwave, use caution. The bowl will be quite hot.

4. Allow the bread to cool slightly before carefully loosening the edges with a paring knife and removing it from the dish, turning it upside down on a paper towel.

5. Make a second loaf of bread using the remaining ingredients. Place aside.

Toasted bread:

6. In a nonstick pan, melt 1 tablespoon of butter. Combine the two slices of bread. Cook until golden brown, about 3 minutes each side, pushing lightly with a spatula to promote even toasting. Place aside.

Make the hollandaise sauce as follows:

7. In a cup fit for the head of an immersion blender, combine the egg yolk, water, lemon juice, and cayenne pepper. I drink from a 16-quart coffee cup.

8. Place the butter in a glass measuring cup, cut into pieces. Melt the butter in 30-second intervals in the microwave.

9. Turn on the immersion blender in the bottom of the cup. Pour the melted butter into the cup while the blender is running. The butter emulsifies with the egg yolk and lemon juice to form a rich, creamy sauce.

Poach the eggs as follows:

10. The simplest method is to use a microwave egg beater and follow the manufacturer's instructions. Typically, a little water is added to the poacher cavities, the eggs are cracked into the poacher, covered, and microwaved for 60-90 seconds for two eggs.

Reheat the Canadian bacon as follows:

11. Place the slices on a microwave-safe dish and microwave for 20 seconds. Alternatively, heat them in the same pan that you used to toast the bread pieces.

Make the eggs Benedict:

12. On each slice of bread, place a slice of Canadian bacon.

13. Include a poached egg.

14. Mix with 2 tablespoons hollandaise sauce. Serve right away.

401kcal | 7g carbs | 20g protein | 32g fat | 16g saturated fat | 990mg sodium | 2g fiber | 2g sugar

PLANT-BASED RECIPES

DELICIOUS EGGPLANT CHIPS

Time to prepare: 10 minutes

Time to cook: 20 minutes

4 servings

INGREDIENTS

- Spray with olive oil

- 2 Japanese eggplants, total weight 35 Oz, unpeeled

- 14 teaspoon ground black pepper 12 teaspoon garlic powder

INSTRUCTIONS

1. Preheat the oven to 450°F. Spray two big nonstick rimmed baking sheets with olive oil spray.

2. Slice the eggplant into 18-inch thick slices using a sharp knife.

3. Arrange the eggplant slices on the prepared baking sheets in a single layer. Drizzle with olive oil and season with black pepper, and garlic powder to taste.

4. Bake the chips for 15 minutes in a preheated oven.

5. Remove from the oven, flip over, spray with additional oil, and bake for another 10-15 minutes*, or until golden brown and crispy.

100kcal | 14g carbohydrate | 2g protein | 5g fat | 287mg sodium | 6g fiber

SPAGHETTI SQUASH FRITTERS

Time to prepare: 10 minutes

Time to cook: 10 minutes

4 servings

INGREDIENTS

- 1 big egg
- 12 tsp black pepper (to taste)
- 1 tablespoon garlic powder
- 18 tsp dried thyme
- 1 cup cooked and well-drained spaghetti squash (6 oz)
- 14 cup blanched almond meal, ground
- 6 cup Parmesan cheese, grated (to taste)
- 2 tbsp. melted butter

INSTRUCTIONS

1. Lightly whisk the egg, black pepper, garlic powder, and thyme in a medium mixing bowl. Combine the pumpkin, almond flour, and Parmesan cheese in a mixing bowl. To combine everything together, use a fork to mix everything together.

2. In a large 12-inch nonstick skillet, melt the butter over medium heat.

3. Pour 14 cup of the spaghetti mixture into the pan for each pancake. Lightly flatten using a spatula. Cook until golden brown on both sides, approximately 3 minutes each side. They are fragile, so handle them with care.

4. Serve immediately, topped with sour cream if preferred.

289kcal | 9g carbohydrate | 11g protein | 24g fat | 10g saturated fat | 524mg sodium | 2g fiber | 3g sugar

ROASTED WHOLE CAULIFLOWER

Time to prepare: 10 minutes

Time to cook: 1h 20 minutes

4 servings

INGREDIENTS

- 1 medium head cauliflower (2 lb. untrimmed)
- 3 tbsp extra-virgin olive oil
- 6 tsp black pepper (to taste)
- 1 tablespoon garlic powder
- 1 paprika teaspoon
- Spray with olive oil

INSTRUCTIONS

1. Preheat the oven to 350°F. In a square baking dish, pour 14 cup of water.

2. Remove the cauliflower's outer leaves but leave the stem intact, cutting it slightly so that the cauliflower head can stand straight in the baking dish (as shown in the video).

3. Wash and dry the cauliflower well with paper towels.

4. Brush the cauliflower with olive oil and season with pepper to taste. Spray olive oil on the seasoned cauliflower.

5. Place the cauliflower head, stem side down, in the preheated baking dish. Cook for 40 minutes, uncovered.

6. Remove the roasting pan from the oven with care, putting it on a mat and leaving the oven on. Transfer the cauliflower to a platter using two broad spatulas. Paper towels should be used to clean the baking sheet (be careful, it is very hot). 14 cup hot water into the baking dish If you're using a Pyrex pan, be sure the water is hot.

7. Place the cauliflower stem side down in the pan. Drizzle with more olive oil. Return the pan to the oven and bake the cauliflower for another 40 minutes, or until the exterior is golden and crisp and the interior is soft and crispy.

8. Allow to rest for 5 minutes before cutting and serving.

173kcal | 11g carbohydrate | 4g protein | 14g fat | 2g saturated fat | 339mg sodium | 5g fiber | 4g sugar

FISH & SEAFOOD

BAKED SALMON MEATBALLS

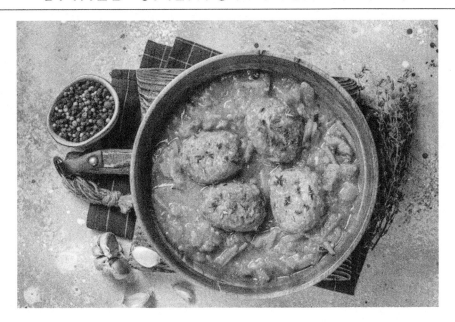

Time to prepare: 15 minutes

Time to cook: 35 minutes

4 servings

INGREDIENTS

- 17 Oz fresh salmon
- 2 eggs
- 2 potatoes
- to taste parsley

- 1 grated organic lemon peel
- to taste breadcrumbs
- to taste extra virgin olive oil
- 10 Oz frozen peas
- 1 large broccoli

PREPARATION

1. Take care of the potatoes: boil them, then peel and mash them with the potato masher. Separately, shred the salmon and add it to the potatoes in a bowl. Mix well until smooth.

2. Add an egg, the parsley you have chopped previously, and the grated organic lemon zest. Continue stirring the mixture, and when it is smooth, create the meatballs.

3. In two plates put, on one side, the other egg that you will have beaten, and on the other the breadcrumbs. Take each meatball and pass it first in the egg, then roll it in the breadcrumbs. When ready, place them in an oven dish, which you will have lightly greased with the help of a kitchen brush.

4. Bake the meatballs at 180° for about 20 minutes, turning them occasionally.

5. Side

6. In a skillet with a drizzle of oil and a little water, cook the frozen peas for about 10 to 15 minutes.

7. Wash and clean the broccoli, then separate the florets from the core. Steam it for about 15 minutes. When it is ready, remove it from the basket.

8. Add a drizzle of oil and serve with the salmon balls while still warm.

287kcal | 2g carbohydrate | 27g protein | 23g fat | 1g saturated fat | 280mg sodium

SALMON SKEWERS WITH VEGETABLES

Time to prepare: 20 minutes

Time to cook: 20 minutes

4 servings

INGREDIENTS

- 12 Oz fresh salmon
- 10 cherry tomatoes
- 2 zucchini
- to taste extra-virgin olive oil
- 12 Oz fresh salad
- 1 lemon

PREPARATION

1. Rinse the salmon under running water and check it for bones. Cut it into cubes of about 3 cm. Sprinkle the salmon with the juice of half a lemon.

2. Also wash the tomatoes and zucchini, cut the latter into slices about 1 cm thick. Compose the skewers by threading the salmon, cherry tomatoes and zucchini slices, alternating the various ingredients.

3. Lay the skewers on a baking sheet covered with baking paper and bake at 175 °C, after lightly peppering the skewers. Bake for 15 minutes (or a few minutes longer if the skewers are not yet ready), turning a couple of times on each side.

4. Meanwhile, wash the salad and dress it with some oil and lemon juice.

5. Serve the skewers warm, accompanied by the salad and dressed with a drizzle of oil.

346kcal | 0.3g carbohydrate | 32g protein | 21g fat | 3g saturated fat | 360mg sodium

BAKED SHRIMP

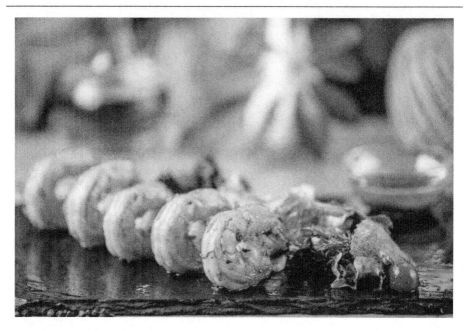

Time to prepare: 10 minutes

Time to cook: 10 minutes

4 servings

INGREDIENTS

- 14 cup raw shelled and hulled shrimp
- 14 cup softened butter (or olive oil)
- 14 tsp black pepper
- 1 tsp. garlic powder
- 12 teaspoon paprika or crushed red pepper
- 14 cup Parmesan cheese, grated

INSTRUCTIONS

1. Preheat the oven to 400°F.

2. Arrange the shrimp on a rimmed baking sheet in a single layer.

3. Toss the shrimp in the melted butter to coat.

4. Sprinkle black pepper, garlic powder, crushed red pepper, and Parmesan cheese over the shrimp.

5. Bake for 8 minutes, or until the shrimp are pink and opaque. To brown the parmesan, place it in the oven for approximately 1 minute.

6. Place the roasted shrimp on a serving plate and drizzle with the cooking juices. Serve right away.

305kcal | 1g carbohydrate | 36g protein | 16g fat | 9g saturated fat | 706mg sodium

SUPER CRAB SALAD

Time to prepare: 15 minutes

Time to cook: 15 minutes

4 servings

INGREDIENTS

- 8 oz of the freshest crabmeat imaginable
- 2 tbsp. red onion, diced
- 2 tbsp. parsley, chopped
- 13 cup mayonnaise
- 1 tsp. Dijon mustard
- 1 tsp spicy chili sauce, such as Frank's Original Cayenne Sauce
- 18 tsp fresh ground black pepper
- 14 teaspoon garlic powder

INSTRUCTIONS

1. Remove the shells from the crabmeat.
2. With a fork, combine the crabmeat, onions, and parsley in a medium mixing basin.
3. Stir in the other ingredients until well combined.

4. Serve right away in a bowl, packed with a tomato or bell pepper, in a lettuce wrap, or over toast, like this almond flour bread.

337kcal | 1g carbohydrate | 19g protein | 27g fat | 4g saturated fat | 846mg sodium | 4g sugar

FISH CHOWDER

Time to prepare: 15 minutes

Time to cook: 15 minutes

4 servings

INGREDIENTS

- 1 tablespoon olive oil
- 1 medium sliced yellow onion (about 1 cup)
- 1 tablespoon fresh garlic, chopped
- 2 cups clam juice or fish broth
- 14 teaspoon ground black pepper
- 1 tablespoon dried thyme
- 14 teaspoon of paprika
- 18 tsp cayenne pepper
- 1 pound cod fillets, skinless and boneless, cut into 2-inch pieces
- 1 quart thick cream
- 4 tablespoons chopped parsley
- 4 tablespoons bacon bits, chopped

INSTRUCTIONS

1.In a large saucepan over medium heat, heat the oil. Cook until the onions are softened, approximately 5 minutes. Cook, stirring constantly, for 1 minute longe

2.Combine pepper, dried thyme, paprika, and cayenne pepper.

3 Pour in the clam juice. Bring to a low heat and bring to a boil.

4.Combine the fish parts. Ensure that they are thoroughly immersed. If not, add a bit extra broth or water.

5.Return the soup to a medium simmer. Cover the saucepan and reduce the heat to low. Simmer for 5-7 minutes, or until the salmon is just cooked through.

6.In the microwave, heat the heavy cream for 60 seconds. Combine it with the soup. Remove from the heat.

7.Ladle the soup into four bowls. Serve garnished with parsley and bacon pieces.

412kcal | 6g carbohydrate | 28g protein | 28g fat | 15g saturated fat | 1417mg sodium | 1g fiber | 3g sugar

DESSERTS

SUPER BANANA DESSERT

Time to prepare: 5 minutes

Time to cook: --

4 servings

INGREDIENTS

- 12 Oz white yogurt
- 2 very ripe bananas
- 1 ripe banana
- 1,7 Oz dark chocolate (optional)
- 2,8 Oz shelled walnuts

PREPARATION

1. Peel two bananas, cut them into rounds and place them in a blender along with the yogurt and walnuts. Blend until the mixture is smooth and homogeneous.

2. Pour the resulting cream into small glasses or jars, in which you will serve it. Slice the remaining banana into rounds and use it to decorate each dessert portion.

3. If desired, grate the dark chocolate and use it as a garnish.

CARROT CAKE

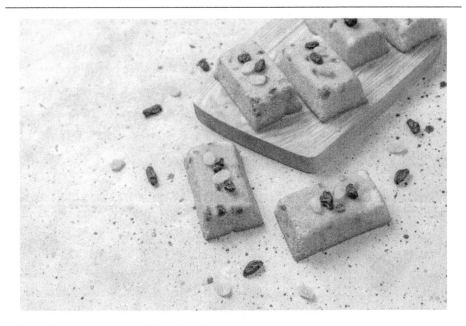

Time to prepare: 20 minutes

Time to cook: 20 minutes

4 servings

INGREDIENTS

- 12 tbsp butter for the pan
- four huge eggs
- 12 c. avocado oil
- 12 cup sugar 1 12 teaspoon stevia glycerite
- 12 cup blanched almond meal, finely ground (6 oz - it is best to measure by weight)

- 2 tablespoons cinnamon powder

- 14 teaspoon ground allspice

- 12 cup finely shredded carrots 1 teaspoon gluten-free baking powder (not excessive amounts)

Cream cheese icing:

- 1 8-ounce box softened cubed cream cheese

- 12 cup powdered sugar 1 12 teaspoon stevia glycerite

- 12 tsp pure vanilla extract

INSTRUCTIONS

1. Preheat the oven to 325°F. Butter an 8-inch square baking pan generously. Alternatively, line it with baking paper and oil it.

2. In a large mixing bowl, combine the eggs, oil, and stevia until well combined.

3. Using a rubber spatula and a hand whisk, combine the almond flour. Whisk until well combined.

4. Combine the cinnamon, allspice, and baking powder in a mixing bowl.

5. Mix in the shredded carrots.

6. Smooth the ingredients into the prepared pan using a rubber spatula. Bake for 25 minutes, or until the cake is fluffy and aromatic and a toothpick inserted into the middle comes out clean.

7. Cold the cake in the pan on a cooling rack for 1 hour, or until totally cool.

8. When the cake has fully cooled, make the frosting by whisking together the soft cream cheese, stevia, and vanilla until creamy and fluffy.

9. To loosen the cake, run a knife over the pan's edges. Make nine squares out of the cake. Slide a cake paddle under each slice and pull it out to remove it from the pan.

10. Divide the icing equally among the cake pieces using a soup spoon. Spread the icing evenly over each slice using a tiny spatula (just as if it were a cupcake).

344kcal | 8g carbohydrate | 9g protein | 32g fat | 7g saturated fat | 235mg sodium | 3g fiber | 3g sugar

YOGURT CAKE

Time to prepare: 15 minutes

Time to cook: 30 minutes

4 servings

INGREDIENTS

- Pan spray with avocado oil
- three huge eggs
- 1 cup plain Greek yogurt (I use Fage 5 percent)
- 12 cup sugar = 1 1/2 tablespoons stevia glycerite
- 1 tbsp. vanilla extract
- 12 cup blanched almond meal, finely ground (6 oz)
- 12 tsp baking soda

INSTRUCTIONS

1. Preheat the oven to 325°F. Coat a 9-inch cake pan liberally with oil.

2. In a medium mixing bowl, combine the eggs, yogurt, stevia, and vanilla.

3. Beat in the almond flour until the mixture is smooth and lump-free.

4. Mix in the baking soda.

5. Transfer the batter to the prepared pan using a rubber spatula.

6. Bake for 30 minutes, or until the top is golden brown and a toothpick inserted into the middle comes out clean.

7. Allow the cake to cool in the pan on a wire rack for 30 minutes before slicing and serving.

186kcal | 6g carbohydrate | 9g protein | 14g fat | 2g saturated fat | 156mg sodium | 3g fiber | 2g sugar

GRILLED PEACHES

Time to prepare: 10 minutes

Time to cook: 15 minutes

4 servings

INGREDIENTS

- 4 medium ripe but firm peaches
- 2 tablespoons melted unsalted butter

INSTRUCTIONS

1. Heat a grill or skillet over medium heat.

2. Cut the peaches in half and remove the stone: With a sharp paring knife, cut each peach in half. Then rotate each half in opposite directions to pull them apart. Use your fingers to remove the stone. If it is stuck, carefully slide the knife under the stone and then pull it away.

3. Brush the peaches all over the surface with melted butter.

4. Place the peaches, cut side down, on the grill. Grill until tender and slightly charred, about 4 minutes per side. Serve immediately.

93kcal | 11g carbohydrate | 1g protein | 6g fat | 3g saturated fat | 1mg sodium | 2g fiber | 8g sugar

BONUS

Dr. Sebi's Alkaline and Anti-Inflammatory Diet for Beginners 2022

Included +600 easy and delicious recipes!

CONCLUSION

Most people would like to eat healthy. And even if you already eat well most of the time, you are likely to want to continue to do so. The benefits of eating well are obvious: you have more energy, your health benefits, and your productivity increases. So, if we want to eat healthy and if it is clear why we should do so, why is it so difficult to eat healthy? More importantly, is there anything we can do to make it easier?

I myself was a disaster at achieving long-term goals. While I was quite good when working on short deadlines, if a project lasted longer than a month my time management was totally inadequate. I suffered because of this, because I felt I was the only one who could not succeed in big goals. Then I started to carefully study people who are good with long-term projects, and my state of mind changed. In fact, I believe that no one is good at long-term goals.

The difference is that in the fact that some people are good at breaking down long-term goals into short-term goals. They work every day or week on a small aspect and at the end of the project, they enjoy this big, beautiful achievement. Good habits -- healthy eating, for example -- work in much the same way. Some people are very good at breaking their long-term goals into small behaviors that they can focus on every day. In other words, they are good at focusing on daily actions rather than the big goals that should enable them to change their lives.

In the end, it is actually these daily actions that turn into powerful habits such that they change lives. And a good habit starts with dividing the ultimate goal into very small steps. I haven't gotten good at long-term goals yet, but I'm getting better. And I have learned a lot along this path. So here is a way to use this methodology to start eating healthy . Good habits are smaller than you think. We are often caught up in the end goal and think we have to achieve it all at once; but it is usually better to start in small steps. Here is a list of what you need to do if you want to eat healthy:

- You need to buy new groceries.

- You need to prepare healthy foods.

- You need to eat healthy food.

- You have to clean and wash dishes.

If you are the kind of person who eats often, then these four steps represent a huge change in your daily life. It is unlikely that you will change all these things at the same time. I think most diets fail not because of a lack of willpower or motivation, but because we don't follow them for long enough. Take a look at that list again. If you're trying to change all these things at the same time, no wonder it's hard to stick to the diet. But imagine a different scenario... What if you eliminated all but the most critical part of the new habit? For example, what would happen if you did these 3 things?

1. Start intermittent fasting. This allows you to eat two healthy meals a day once or twice a week instead of three.

2. For the first two months of the diet, buy disposable dishes to minimize clean-up time.

3. For the first month, buy ready-to-eat food 5 times a week at some deli or organic restaurant (there are now many online at attractive prices). This would ensure that you eat healthy when you get home from work in the evening without having to cook.

Now, I realize that buying disposable plates and ordering food is expensive, but we are not talking about doing it forever. We're just talking about making it an easier habit to start. We're talking about making an investment for the first couple of months to make it as easy as possible to start eating healthy. With the pattern above, the only thing you have to do each month is eat healthy meals. In the second month, you will start buying healthier groceries and cooking your own meals. In the third month, you will stop buying disposable dishes and do the complete cleanse. Imagine how much easier it will be to eat healthy when you remove some initial barriers.

Of course, you can adapt this strategy to your needs. If you can't afford to buy ready-made, healthy food for 5 meals a week, how about 2 meals a week? Do whatever suits you, but the general idea is to eliminate everything but the most important task. Break the goal down into smaller parts, eliminate excuses and make it as easy as possible to say yes to your new habit. You don't have to do everything, you just have to start doing it. It may require an investment, but answer honestly: would you rather simplify the process, pay a little more now and stick to a healthy diet or try to do it all at once, exhaust your willpower and give vent to your frustration as early as two weeks later? If you are going to consider a major long-term change, know that smaller is better, especially in the beginning.

Best Regards,

Serena Stewart

Printed in Great Britain
by Amazon

24450315R00069